22 HEALING ACUPRESSURE POINTS

FAST EASY GUIDE TO NATURAL HEALING

KARL SWOPE DC

Karl Swope, *22 Healing Acupressure Points: Fast Easy Guide to Natural Healing* Copyright © 2014 by Karl Swope.

Interior design by Leslie Monroe
Printed in the United States of America

ISBN: 1499783515

ISBN-13: 978-1499783513

DEDICATION

To my wife,
daughter and granddaughter,
you made this book possible.

CONTENTS

INTRODUCTION

I have tried to make a book that is practical for everyone. You do not need to be a healthcare professional to help yourself, your friends and family to feel better.

Acupressure with your fingers is just like acupuncture with needles, in that you are stimulating acupuncture points to cause the body to respond in a positive manner.

The beauty of acupressure is that it is very safe and these 22 points are "normalizing" points. That means if the body needs to be stimulated, stimulation results from pressure to the point. If the body needs to be sedated, sedation is the result. You may ask, " How does that work?" The short answer is, I do not know. What I do know from 30 years of working with Trigger points, Acupressure points and Reflexology points is that you can only help the person, you can not make things worse.

As a chiropractic student I was having a very bad flare up of my old low back injury. I was being adjusted 6-7 times per day just to try to sit in class and learn how to become a chiropractor. It hit me, "If Chiropractic can not get me me out of pain, why am I spending all this money to learn it?"

I needed to seriously rethink my career choice. A group of my friends and I started to explore every alternative treatment we could find. We took classes outside of school in Thai massage, Reflexology, Shiatsu massage, Reiki, Kinesiology, Acupuncture and Trigger point Therapy. We finally came up with a treatment plan that allowed me to go for two weeks between adjustments.

I knew Chiropractic could help myself and others but it needed to be coupled with other therapies, in order to treat the whole person. In my thirst for knowledge of how to help others, I went so far as to become eligible to sit for the California State Exam in Acupuncture. We learned how to help our patients using Chiropractic and alternative therapies to bring them back to a state of health and well being, not one of disease.

To help my patients I put together lists of the most powerful points and what they treat. You have just purchased a culmination of 30 years of work and probably 3500 hours of study, in one little book.

We are going to look at these points like switches. If you turn this switch, this will happen. Usually. Will it always happen? No, because, like a light switch, sometimes the bulb is burnt out. Sometimes the circuit breaker is off. Sometimes the whole neighborhood is without power. When that happens, no amount of stimulation to these points is going to work. You need to call the professionals like me and let them evaluate you and treat accordingly.

Disclaimer: Do not apply pressure to an injured area. If you try to push on one of these points and the person has a cut, a bruise or a broken bone, at that site, take appropriate action. Clean cuts and bandage. Don't push on bruised tissue, and get professional help for broken bones. Above all use common sense.

HOW TO USE THIS BOOK

There are two indexes in the back of the book. One is by body part. IE. If your head hurts, use the points for head and neck. The other is by ailment. IE. If you have sinusitis, follow the points for sinusitis.

You should press hard on the points as long as you can stand the discomfort. When working on others ask them to say stop when it hurts too much. For some people this will be very light pressure, for others, very deep.

Press each point about 10 - 15 seconds. Treat them as often as you wish, ***but do not create bruises***.

You will find one page for each point. The page numbers are intentionally lined up for ease of use.

NOTE: Follow the order of the points listed under the conditions. IE. Constipation, 9,15,1,8,14. Do number 9 first then 15 etc. Do not go in numerical order.

DEFINITIONS

TMF: Time of Maximum Function

TSUN (Pronounced tsoon): Relative Body Unit

1 tusn – thumb width   3 tusn – 4 fingers

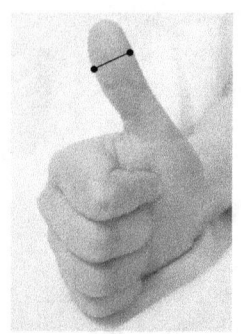 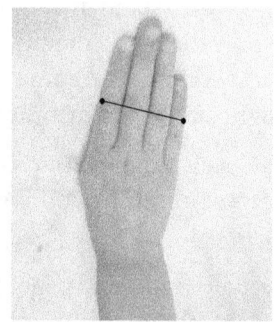

1.5 tusn – knuckle to knuckle or 2 fingers

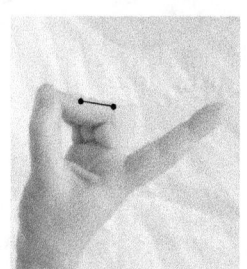 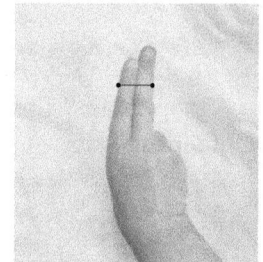

ACUPRESSURE POINT 1

Name: Large Intestine 4 (LI-4)
Treats: **Face, Head**

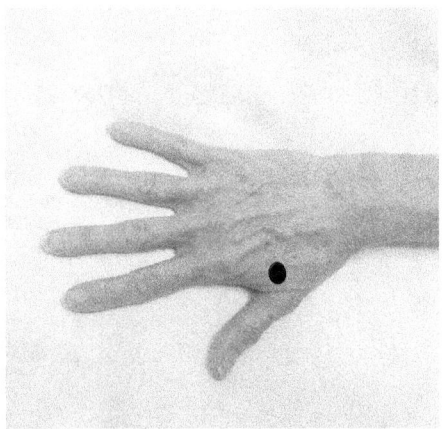

Location:

Point is located where the first and second metacarpals intersect on the back of the hand.

Helpful Hints:

Press your thumb against your first finger and you will see a bump beside the thumb. Push straight in towards the index finger and you will trap the point. Or simply pinch the web between your thumb and first finger.

TMF: 5-7 AM

ACUPRESSURE POINT 2

Name: Lung 7 (L-7)

Treats: **Neck**

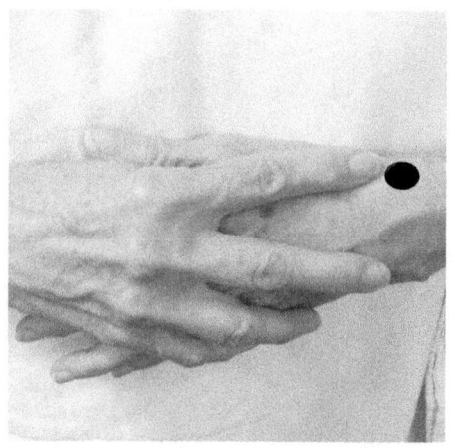

Location:

Point is located 1 ½ tsun toward the elbow on the radial edge of the wrist.

Helpful Hints:

Hook thumbs together and the top index finger will rest on the pint on the radius bone.

TMF: 3-5AM

ACUPRESSURE POINT 3

Name: Pericardium (circulation sex) 6 (P-6)

Treats: **Chest**

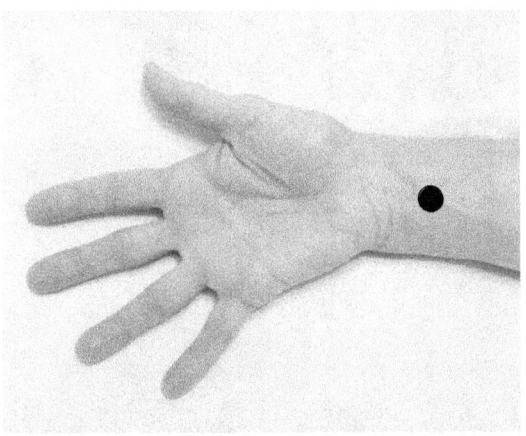

Location:

Point is located 2 tsun toward the elbow in the medial position between the tendons.

Helpful Hints:

Two finger widths (proximal) above the crease in the wrist on the inside of the arm.

TMF: 7-9PM

3

ACUPRESSURE POINT 4

Name: Lung 5 (L-5)

Treats: **Respiratory System**

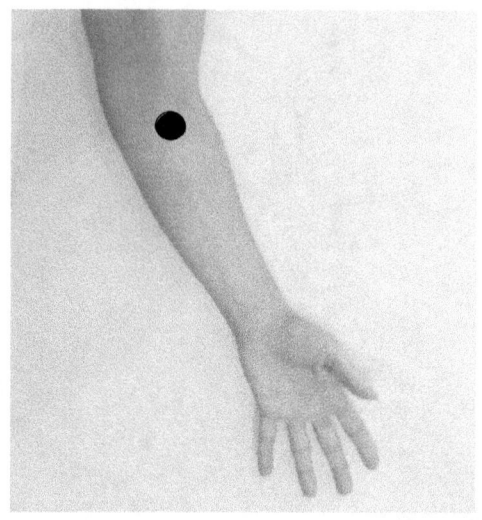

Location:

Point is located in the crease of the elbow.

Helpful Hints:

At the crease in the elbow where the head of the radius articulates with the humorous.

TMF: 3-5AM

ACUPRESSURE POINT 5

Name: Large Intestine 11 (LI-11)

Treats: **Arm, Skin**

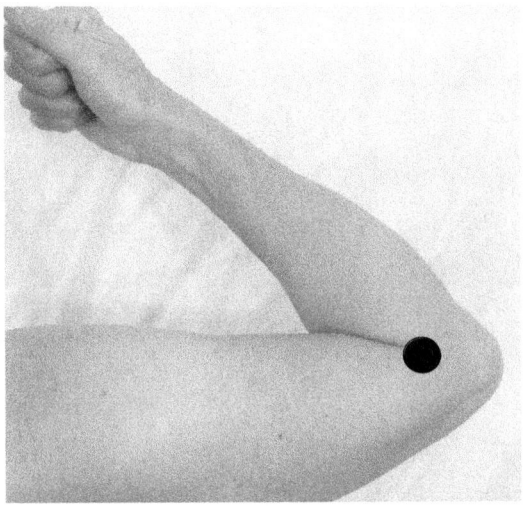

Location:

Point is located on the arm when bent at the end of the crease in the elbow.

Helpful Hints:

Hand should face upwards and trap the point at the end of crease against the elbow.

TMF: 5-7AM

ACUPRESSURE POINT 6

Name: Endocrine (Triple Heater) 5 (TH-5)

Treats: **Ear, Hand**

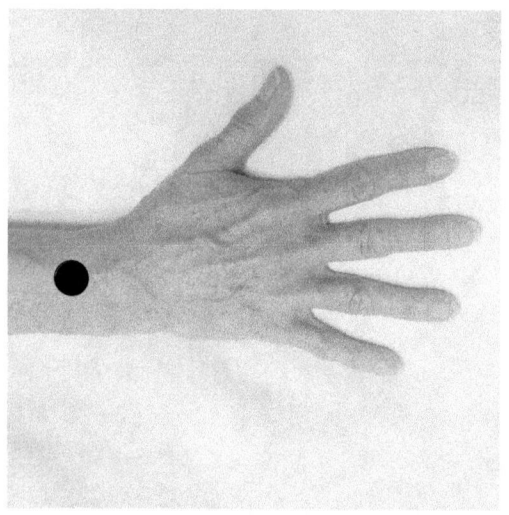

Location:

Point is located 2 tsun toward the elbow in the medial position on the back of the arm from the wrist.

Helpful Hints:

This is opposite of point number 3. Two finger widths (proximal) above the crease in the wrist.

TMF: 9-11 PM

ACUPRESSUREPOINT 7

Name: Heart 7 (H-7)

Treats: **Emergency: Heart and Anxiety**

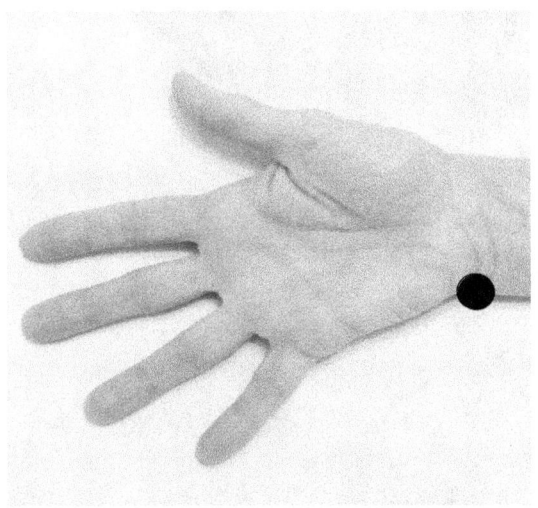

Location:

Point is located on the wrist crease in the hollow directly in line with the fifth metatarsal.

Helpful Hints:

Turn palm to face you; find the hollow directly in line with the pinky-finger.

TMF: 11 AM-1 PM

ACUPRESSUREPOINT 8

Name: Endocrine (Triple Heater) 1 (TH-1)

Treats: **Emergency for Heart Attacks**

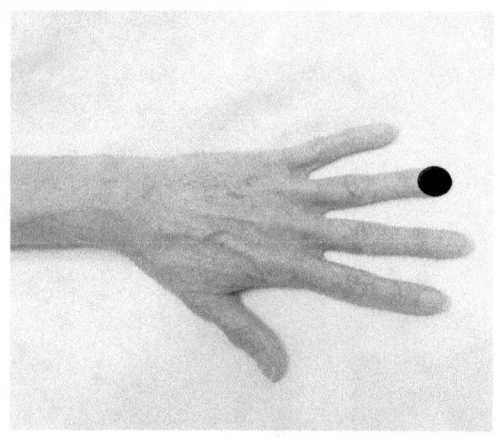

Location:

Point is in the nail bed of the ring finger.

Helpful Hints:

You can bite on this point. It is taught to police in China to treat heart attack victims.

ACUPRESSUREPOINT 9

Name: Stomach 36 (St-36)

Treats: **Upper Abdomen, Energizing**

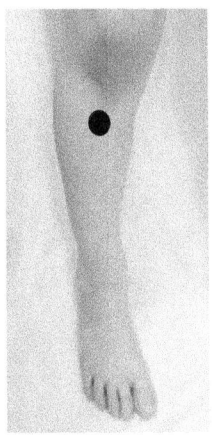

Location:

From the knee 3 tsun down and 1 tsun over.

Helpful Hints:

Cradle the patella with your thumb and forefinger, your middle finger rests on the point.

TMF: 7-9 AM

Caution: Do not over work late in the evening, or you may not sleep well.

ACUPRESSURE POINT 10

Name: Spleen 6 (Sp-6)

Treats: **Lower Abdomen**

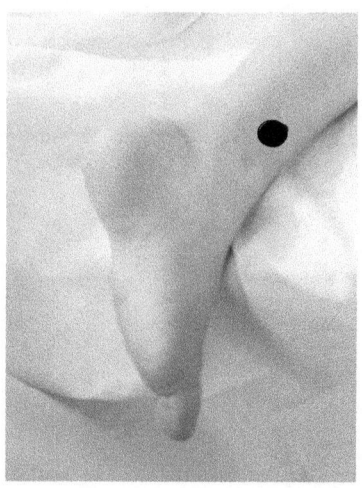

Location:

Point is located 3 tsun above the medial malleolus just behind the tibia.

Helpful Hints:

Three finger widths above the inner ankle-bone.

TMF: 9-11 AM

Caution: Do not over stimulate during pregnancy!

ACUPRESSURE POINT 11

Name: Urinary Bladder 40 (UB-40)

Treats: **Lower Back, Legs**

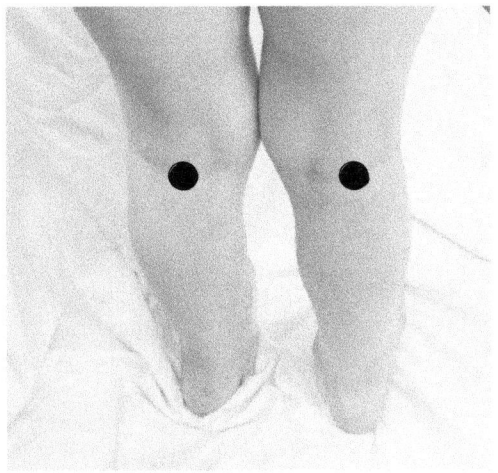

Location:

Point is located behind the knee, right in the middle of the popliteal fossa.

Helpful Hints:

Behind the knee, right in the middle.

TMF: 3-5 PM

Caution: If you feel a pulse, **DO NOT PUSH ON ARTERIES.**

ACUPRESSURE POINT 12

Name: Urinary Bladder 60 (UB-60)

Treats: **Upper Back, Feet, Legs**

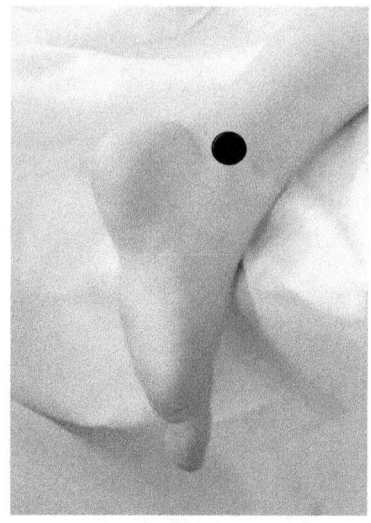

Location:

Point is located ½ tsun behind the lateral malleolus.

Helpful Hints:

One finger width behind the outside of the anklebone.

TMF: 3-5 PM

ACUPRESSURE POINT 13

Name: Liver 3 (Liv-3)
Treats: **Nervous System**

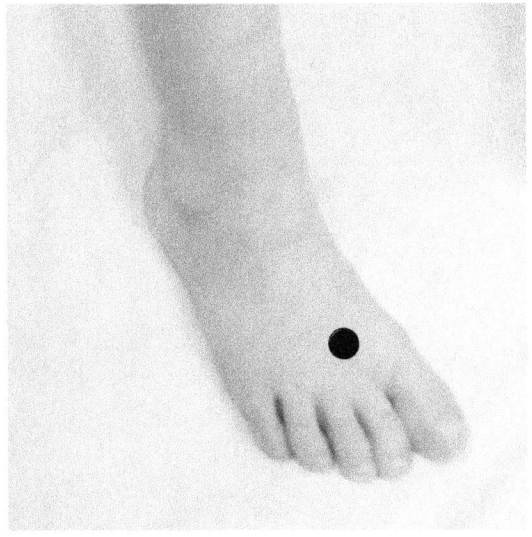

Location:

Point is located 1 ½ tsun above the crease between the first and second metatarsals.

Helpful Hints:

Two finger widths above the crease between the big and the first toe in the web of the foot. On top of the foot.

TMF: 1-3 AM

ACUPRESSURE POINT 14

Treats: **Maxillary Sinuses**

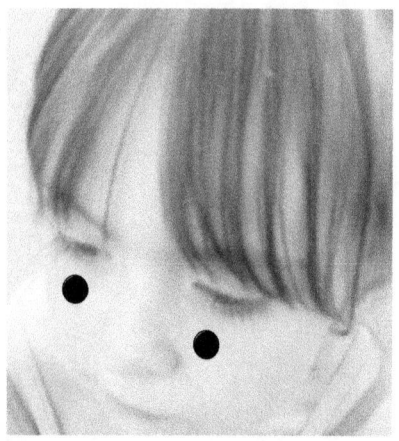

Location:

Points are below the eyes on the maxillary bone, on either side of the nose.

Helpful Hints:

Use your thumbs when working on yourself. (Like junior birdman) On someone else it's best to stand behind them to allow them to rest their head against your chest.

ACUPRESSURE POINT 15

Treats: **Headaches, Sinuses, and General Well being.**

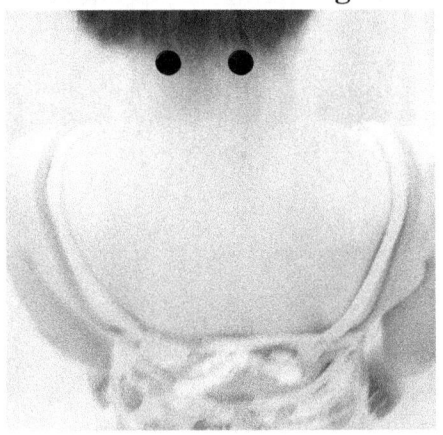

Location:

Where the neck muscles join the skull and in-between.

Helpful Hints:

Cup the head with hands and place thumbs on either side of the spine. Work all around this area to find the most tender spots, then treat.

ACUPRESSURE POINT 16

Name: Gall Bladder 34 (GB-34)

Treats: **Knees, Legs, Muscles, Tendons**

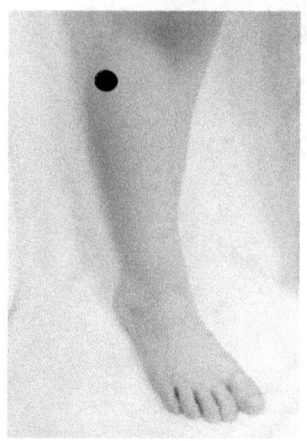

Location:

Point is located 2 tsun behind point 8 on the head of the fibula.

Helpful Hints:

Cup the kneecap and the small finger rests on the hollow.

TMF: 11 PM - 1 AM

ACUPRESSURE POINT 17

Name: Conception Vessel 12 (CV-12)

Treats: **Upper Abdomen**

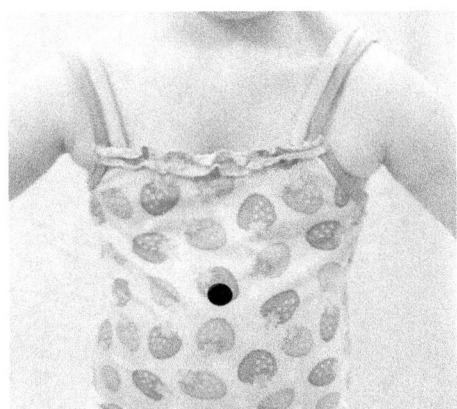

Location:

Point is located halfway between the navel and the sternum.

Helpful Hints:

Located in the middle of the stomach.

Tip: The CV points can be used to treat all abdominal ailments at the level of the organ that has the problem. I.E. heart = midline at the level of the heart etc.

Caution: If you feel a pulse, **DO NOT PUSH ON ARTERIES**. Here, you are near the bifurcation of the Aorta.

ACUPRESSURE POINT 18

Name: Conception Vessel 6 (CV-6)

Treats: **Lower Abdomen**

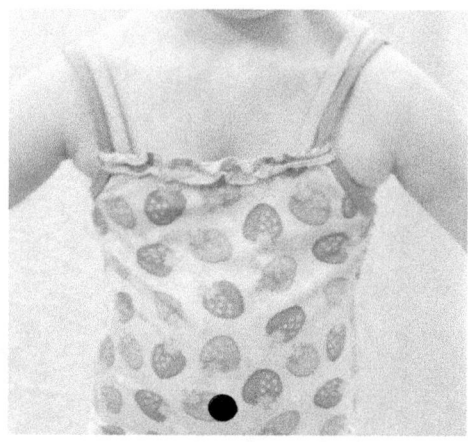

Location:

Point is located 1 ½ tsun below navel.

Helpful Hints:

Two fingers below belly button.

Tip:

The CV points can be used to treat all abdominal ailments at the level of the organ that has the problem. I.E. heart = midline at the level of the heart etc.

ACUPRESSURE POINT 19

Name:Urinary Bladder 11 (UB-11)

Treats: **Back, Bones, Neck, Shoulders**

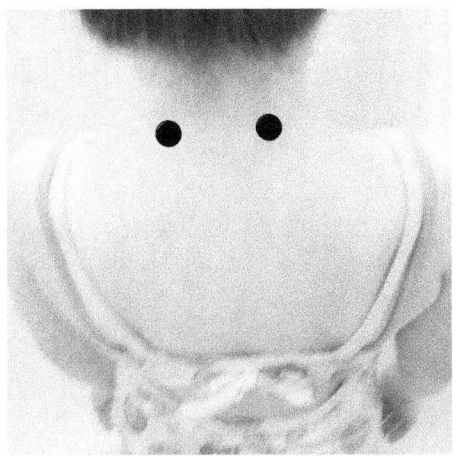

Location:

Point is located on the back, 1 ½ tsun from the spine level with the top of the shoulders.

Helpful Hints:

Best found by someone else. With their hands on your shoulders, the point is where their thumbs come to rest on either side of the spine. This is about where UB points are located.

TMF: 3-5 PM

ACUPRESSURE POINT 20

Name: Urinary Bladder 17 (UB-17)

Treats: **Blood, Heart, Skin**

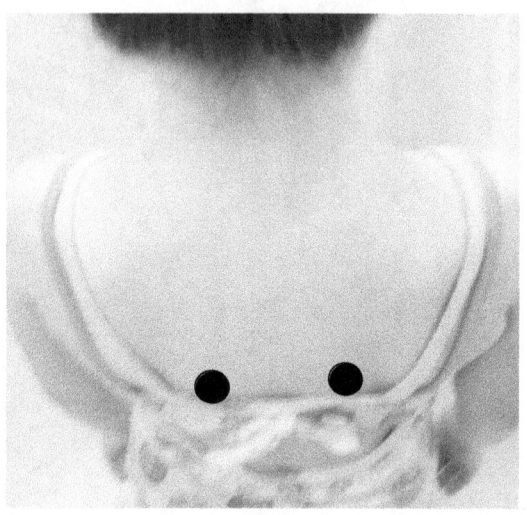

Location:

Point is located below the scapula, 1 ½ tsun from the spine.

Helpful Hints:

Best found by someone else. Point is on either side of the spine below the shoulder blades. Directly below point 19.

TMF: 3-5 PM

ACUPRESSURE POINT 21

Name: Governing Vessel 26 (GV-26)

Treats: **Emergency for Unconsciousness,
Lower Back**

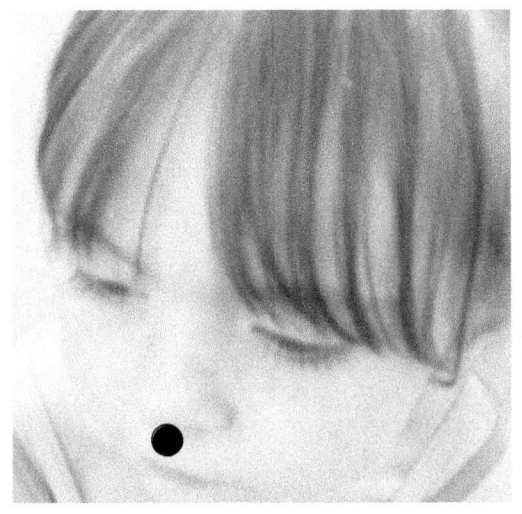

Location:

Point is located on the philtrum.

Helpful Hints:

Above the center of the upper lip.

ACUPRESSURE POINT 22

Treats: **Sinuses**

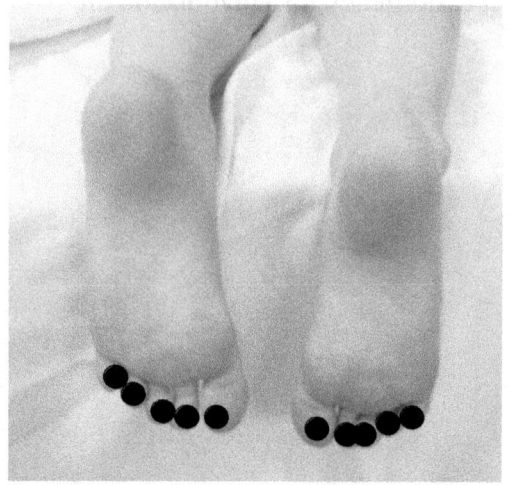

Location:

Points are in the pads of the toes.

Helpful Hints:

Place thumb on the nail bed, and index finger on the pads of the toes, then squeeze firmly.

EMERGENCY POINTS

Anxiety   7, 8

Bleeding 20, 9

Convulsions 21, 1, 7, 8

Cramping:

    Calf 12, 11

    Foot 12

    Hand 1, 6

    Leg 12

    Menstrual 18, 10

Depression 13, 3, 9

Fainting 21

Fear 2, 13

Heart Attack 8

Hysteria 3, 21, 7, 8

Motion Sickness 17, 3

Toothache 1

Vertigo 1, 6, 9

POINTS FOR HEALING
BY AILMENT

Abdominal Pain:

    Lower 10, 18, 1

    Upper 9, 17

Acne 20, 5

Addictions:

    Drugs 13

    Food 17, 9, 3

    Tobacco 2

Allergies 20, 1, 5, 9, 10

Amnesia 1, 13, 9

Anxiety 17, 13, 9

Anxiety with palpitations 7, 3, 8,13

Apoplexy 1, 9, 21, 4

Appetite (deficient or excessive) 9, 17

Arteriosclerosis 20, 9, 1, 10, 8

Arthritis (see body part) 19, 1, 9, 10

Asthma 4, 2, 3

Bleeding,Blood Diseases 20, 9

Breathing 3, 9, 4

Bronchitis 3, 4, 9, 19

Bursitis:

>Knee 12, 16

>Shoulder 5

Childbirth   10   **CAUTION: DO NOT STIMULATE DURING PREGNANCY!**

Cholera 1, 17, 9, 4

Coccyx 11

Common Cold 1, 9, 2, 3

Colitis 10, 18, 9

Concussion 1, 2

Convulsions 1, 8, 3, 5, 7

Cough 4, 2, 3, 1, 17

Cramping:

>Calf 12, 11

>Foot 12

>Hand 1, 6

>Leg 12

>Menstrual 18, 10

Cerebral Vascular Accident 1, 9, 21, 4

Cystitis 18, 10

Deafness 1, 6

Depression 13, 3, 9

Diabetes 10, 9, 3, 18, 20

Digestive Trouble 10, 9, 3, 1, 17

Dizziness 6, 17, 9, 1

Jaundice 13, 9, 17, 20

Joint Pain 17, 8, 13, 20

Laryngitis 4, 2

Lingual Paralysis 7, 1, 8

Lumbago 11, 21, 12

Mastitis 13, 3

Meniere's Syndrome1, 9, 6

Menstruation:

    Cramping 10, 18

    Excessive 10, 18, 13, 1

    Insufficient 10, 18, 13, 1, 9

    Painful 10 18, 13, 1

Menopause 18, 1, 10,9

Mental Illness 7, 9, 8, 1, 17,10

Metritis 10, 18

Migraine Headache 1, 17, 10, 9, 18, 15

Motion Sickness 17, 1, 6, 9, 3

Mumps 1, 6, 9

Muscle Spasm 14

Nausea 17, 3, 10

Nephritis 10

Nervous Anxiety with Palpitations 7, 13, 9

Nervousness 13, 9

Neuralgia;

    Back, Lower 11, 21, 13

    Back, Upper 12, 19, 13

    Face 1, 9, 13, 15

    Intercostal 3, 12

    Joint 19

    Limb, Lower 12, 16, 13

    Limb, Upper 5, 1, 6, 3, 2, 19, 13

Neck 2, 5, 12, 13

Neurasthenia 13, 1, 9, 18

Night Sweats 3, 10

Nocturia 10, 18

Nosebleed 1, 15

Otitis (ear ache) 1, 6

Overeating 17, 9, 3

Paralysis (see body part) 16, 10, 6, 1, 9

Phlebitis 20, 9

Pleurisy 4, 2, 9, 3, 19, 8

Pneumonia 3, 4, 19

Premature Ejaculation 10, 18

Prostatitis 10, 18

Pruritis Vulvae 18, 10

Renal Disorders 10, 9

Rhinitis 1

Rubella 1

Unconsciousness 21, 10, 17

Urinary Disorder 10, 18

Vaginitis 10, 18

Varicose Veins 20

Vertigo 1, 6, 9

Vomiting 17, 9, 1, 10, 3, 20

Well Being 15

Whiplash 2, 5, 12, 19, 15

Wrist Pain 6, 1, 5

POINTS FOR HEALING BY BODY PART

Abdomen:

    Lower 10, 18

    Upper 9, 17

Ankle 12

Anus 1, 10

Arm 5, 1, 4

Back:

    Lower 11, 21

    Upper 12

Bladder 10, 18

Blood 20

Bones 19

Bowels 10

Brain 1, 13

Breast 3, 13

Buttock 11, 16

Cheeks 1

Chest 3, 2

Coccyx 11 12

Colon 1, 10, 18

Ear 6, 1

Elbow 5

Esophagus 1, 3

Eye 1

Face 1

Fallopian Tube 18, 10

Finger 1, 6

Foot 12

Forehead 1

Gall Bladder 9, 17

Genital-Urinary System 10, 18

Gums 1

Hair 11

Hand 6, 1, 3

Head 1, 15, 14

Heart 7, 3, 8

Hip 12, 11

Intestines 1, 10, 18

Jaw 1

Kidney 10

Knee 11, 12, 16

Large Intestine 10, 18

Leg 11, 12 10

Limb 9

Stomach 9, 17, 3

Teeth 1

Testicle 18, 10

Thigh 12, 11

Throat 1, 4, 3

Toe 12

Tongue 1

Tonsil 1, 4, 5

Trachea 1, 2

Ureter 10, 18

Urethra 10, 18

Urinary Bladder 10, 18

Vagina 10, 18

Wrist 6, 1, 5

ABOUT THE AUTHOR

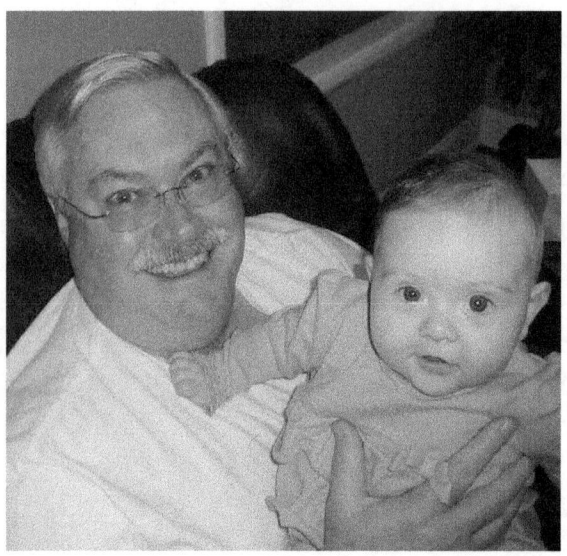

Karl Swope is a doctor of Chiropractic, husband and father. He graduated from the Los Angeles College of Chiropractic, where he discovered the power of Acupuncture for himself. Since then he as has been on a mission to help others, and teach his passion for healing. He loves to fish, watch baseball, and play with his grandchildren.